Acupuncture

The Natural Ways to do Acupressure Effectively to Treat Yourself

Keyile Martins

Copyright © 2020 Keyile Martins

All rights reserved. No part of this publication may be reproduced, distributed, or transmitted in any form or by any means, including photocopying, recording, or other electronic or mechanical methods, without the prior written permission of the publisher, except in the case of brief quotations embodied in critical reviews and specific other non-commercial uses permitted by copyright law.

ISBN: 978-1-63750-175-7

Table of Contents

ACUPUNCTURE 1

INTRODUCTION 5

CHAPTER 1 6

   How Does Acupuncture Work? 6
   Uses of Acupuncture 6
   Great things about Acupuncture 7
      Side Effects of Acupuncture 12
      Does Acupuncture Harm? 13

CHAPTER 2 15

   6 Pressure Factors for Anxiety Relief 15
   Know when to see a Medical Expert 22
      Acupuncture for Anxiety Attacks 23
      Getting Treated with Acupuncture 26
      The 5 Best Acupuncture Factors for Anxiety 27

CHAPTER 3 32

   The Acupuncture Factors for Legs 32
   Acupuncture & Hormone Balance 35

CHAPTER 4 39

   Cluster Headaches 39
   Characteristics of Cluster Headaches 40
   Symptoms 42
      Possible Causes and Triggers 43

CHAPTER 5 48

   How to use Pressure Factors to alleviate Headaches 48

CHAPTER 6 52

   Acupuncture for Digestive Problems 52
   The Sources of Digestive Disorders 54
   Acupuncture and Abdomen Disorders 55

CHAPTER 7 .... **60**

ACUPUNCTURE FOR LOWERING HIGH BLOOD PRESSURE 60

ACUPUNCTURE AND STROKE 63

Dangers and Warnings 67

Alternatives to Acupuncture 68

CHAPTER 8 .... **70**

HEALTH ADVANTAGES OF HEARING ACUPUNCTURE 70

USES 70

BENEFITS 72

Using Hearing Acupuncture for Health 75

Introduction

Did you ever wonder how acupuncture works? This book strips away the mystery. Each acupuncture point has unique functions, which are explained in plain English for the non-acupuncturist.

How to do acupressure effectively to treat yourself. This book explains which points are the best to treat different ailments. Acupuncture treats pain, stress, fatigue, emotional disorders, insomnia, digestive problems, and many internal disorders.

Acupuncturists place hair-thin needles to specific acupuncture factors throughout your body to revive the movement of qi, balance the body's energy, stimulate curing, and promote rest.

Relating to TCM theory, there are over 1000 acupuncture factors on your body, each laying on a low profile energy route, or "meridian"; each meridian is associated with a different body organ system.

Chapter 1

How Does Acupuncture Work?

Acupuncture functions by stimulating the discharge of endorphins, your body's natural pain-relieving chemicals, it also affects the autonomic nervous system and the release of chemicals that regulate blood circulation and pressure, reduces swelling, and calm the mind.

Uses of Acupuncture

Acupuncture is reported to be useful in addressing several health issues, including:

- Anxiety.

- Arthritis.

- Persistent pain (such as headaches, back pain, neck pain).

- Depression.

- Insomnia.

- Migraines.

- Nausea.

- Sciatica.

- Sinus congestion.

- Anxiety and stress.

- Tinnitus.

- Weight loss

Some individuals use acupuncture to market fertility. Cosmetic acupuncture, also called facial acupuncture, is utilized to enhance the appearance of skin.

Great things about Acupuncture

Some results from the available research on the advantages of acupuncture are:

- **Low Back Pain**

For a written report published in the history of *Internal Medicine in 2017*, experts published the analyzed trials on the utilization of non-pharmacologic therapies (including acupuncture) for low back pain; the report authors discovered that acupuncture was associated with reduced pain strength and better function soon after the acupuncture treatment, weighed against no acupuncture.

- **Migraines**

In 2016 review, released in the *Cochrane Database of Systematic Reviews*, researchers examined 22 previously released trials (involving 4985 individuals); within their summary, they discovered that adding acupuncture to the treating migraine symptoms may decrease the rate of recurrence; nevertheless, the size of the result is small in comparison with a sham acupuncture treatment.

- **Tension Headaches**

A 2016 review (involving 12 tests and 2349 individuals) shows that acupuncture involving at least six sessions can help people with regular tension of headaches. The analysts note that the precise factors used during treatment may play a less important role than previously thought, which most of the power may be credited to needling results.

- **Knee Pain**

An analysis of previous post studies discovered that acupuncture improved physical function in people who have chronic knee pain, credited to osteoarthritis, but it seemed to provide only short-term (up to 13 weeks) pain relief.

Another review, posted in JAMA Surgery, analyzed non-pharmacological interventions for pain management after total knee arthroplasty and found evidence that acupuncture delayed the utilization of patient-controlled use of opioid medication to alleviate pain.

A Typical Acupuncture Treatment is similar to the initial appointment; you'll be asked to complete health history; the acupuncturist starts the visit by requesting about your wellbeing, diet, rest, stress level, and other lifestyle practices. You might be asked about your feelings, appetite, food needs and wants, and response to changes in heat and cold seasons.

Throughout your visit, the acupuncturist will test your appearance carefully, taking note of your tone, tone of voice, and tongue color and covering. He or she will need your pulse at three factors on each wrist, noting the power, quality, and tempo. In Chinese medication, the tongue and pulses are believed to reflect the fitness of your body organ systems and meridians.

Typically, acupuncture uses 6 to 15 tiny needles per treatment (the number of needles doesn't indicate the intensity of the procedure). The needles should be left for 10 to 20 minutes; the acupuncturist may twist the needles for added impact.

Your acupuncturist could use additional techniques throughout your program, including:

Moxibustion: this can also be known as "moxa," moxibustion entails the utilization of warmed sticks (created from dried out herbs) held close to the acupuncture needles to warm and stimulate the acupuncture factors.

Cupping: Glass mugs are put on your skin so that there

can be a suction impact. In TCM theory, cupping can be used to alleviate the stagnation of qi and bloodstream.

Herbs: Chinese natural herbs may be gotten by from teas, pills, and pills.

Electro-acupuncture: A powerful device is linked to two to four acupuncture needles, providing a weak electric current that stimulates the acupuncture needles through the treatment.

Laser acupuncture: this is used to activate acupuncture factors without the utilization of needles.

Ear acupuncture, also called auricular acupuncture, may also be used through the treatment for weight reduction, smoking cessation, addictions, and anxiety.

Although the space of the acupuncture session may differ from a few moments to over one hour, the regular treatment length is 20 to 30 minutes; the first visit might take up to 60 minutes. Following the treatment, many people feel calm (or even sleepy), while some feel energetic; if you experience any uncommon symptoms, you should seek advice from your doctor.

Side Effects of Acupuncture

Much like any treatment, acupuncture will pose some dangers like bleeding and pains immediately, and the acupuncture needles are inserted. Other undesirable effects can include pores and skin rashes, allergies, bruising, pain, blood loss, nausea, dizziness, fainting, or attacks.

To be able to reduce the threat of serious undesirable effects, acupuncture should be administered with a certified and properly trained practitioner using sterile, disposable needles. According to a written report published in *Scientific Reviews*, acupuncture can cause undesirable severe effects, such as attacks, nerve and blood vessel injuries, problems from needle breakage or remnant needle items, punctured organs, central nervous system or spinal-cord injury,

hemorrhage, and other organ and cells injuries leading to loss of life. Punctured pleural membranes around the lungs can result in collapsed lungs. People who have a unique, anatomical variance known as sternal foramen (an opening in the breastbone) are in threat of lung or center (pericardium) puncture.

There were some reports of needles being left in following the treatment; a written statement released in the *Bulletin of the World Health Business* summarized the acupuncture-related undesirable effects in Oriental studies. Acupuncture might not be right for individuals with specific health issues; the chance of blood loss or bruising raises if you have a blood loss disorder or are taking bloodstream thinners, such as warfarin (Coumadin).

Does Acupuncture Harm?

You might feel hook sting, pinch, ache, or some pain when the acupuncture needle is inserted; some acupuncturists change the acupuncture needle after it's been placed in the torso, by twirling or revolving the needle, moving it along, or utilizing a machine with a little electric pulse or current. Some acupuncturists consider the production of tingling, numbness, heavy feeling, or ache (known as "de qi") desired in attaining the therapeutic impact.

In the event whereby you experience pain, numbness, or pain through the treatment, you should notify your acupuncturist immediately.

Chapter 2

6 Pressure Factors for Anxiety Relief

Understanding anxiety

A lot of people experience stress in their everyday life; you may experience moderate symptoms when facing a challenging or nerve-racking situation. You could also have significantly more severe, long-lasting symptoms that impact your lifestyle, including:

- Feelings of stress, dread, or worry.

- Restlessness.

- Difficulty concentrating.

- Difficulty drifting off to sleep or staying asleep.

- Fatigue.

- Irritability.

- Nausea, headaches, or digestive concerns.

- Feeling too little control.

- Muscle tension.

Anxiety is usually treated with therapy, medication, or a mixture of both. There are also several treatments, including acupressure, which will help.

Acupressure is a kind of traditional Chinese medication that might provide temporary rest from panic symptoms; it requires stimulating pressure factors within you, either by yourself or by using a professional.

Six pressure factors you can test for anxiety alleviation.

1. ***Hall of impression point***

The hall of impression point lies **in the middle of your eyebrows**; applying pressure up to now is thought to assist with both anxiety and stress.

To utilize this point:

- Sit comfortably; it can benefit you to close your eye also.

- Touch the location in the middle of your eyebrows with your index finger or thumb.

- Take decrease, deep breaths, and apply gentle, company pressure in a round movement for 5 to ten minutes.

2. *Heavenly gate point*

The heavenly gate point is situated *in the top shell of your ear*, at the end of the triangle-like hollow there. Stimulating this aspect is said to help relieve anxiousness, stress, and insomnia.

To utilize this point:

- Locate the idea in your ear; it could help use a reflection.

- Apply company, gentle pressure in a round motion for just two minutes.

3. *Make well point*

The shoulder well point is within *your shoulder muscle*. To think it pinches your muscle with your middle finger and thumb. This pressure point is said to assist with relieving stress, muscle tension, and headaches. Additionally, it may stimulate labor, so don't utilize this point if you're pregnant.

To utilize this point:

- Find the idea on your make muscle.

- Pinch the muscle with your thumb and middle finger.

- Apply gentle, firm pressure with your index finger and massage the idea for four to five seconds.

- Release the pinch as you therapeutic massage the point.

4. **Union valley point**

You find this pressure point in **the middle of your thumb and index finger**. Stimulating this aspect is thought to reduce stress, headaches, and neck pain. Just like the shoulder wellpoint, additionally, it may induce labor, so avoid this aspect if you're pregnant.

To utilize this point:

- Together with your index finger and thumb, apply firm pressure to the webbing between your thumb and index finger of your other hand.

- Massage the pressure point for four to five seconds, taking decrease, deep breaths.

5. *Great surge point*

The fantastic surge pressure point is **on your foot**, about several finger widths below the intersection of your big toe and second toe; the idea is based on the hollow right above the bone.

This pressure point can help to lessen anxiety and stress; you can even utilize it for pain, insomnia, and menstrual cramps.

To utilize this point:

- Find the idea by moving your finger down along from in the middle of your first two toes.

- Apply company, deep pressure to the idea.

- Therapeutic massage for four to five mere seconds.

6. *Internal frontier gate point*

You'll find the inner frontier gate point **on your arm**, around three finger widths below your wrist. Stimulating this aspect may help to lessen stress and anxiety, also reducing nausea and pain.

To utilize this point:

- Turn one hand so your palm faces up.
- Together with your other hand, measure three hands below your wrist. The idea is situated here, in the hollow between your tendons.

Apply pressure to the idea and therapeutic massage for four to five seconds.

The study behind acupressure for anxiety

There's limited research about the utilization of acupressure and pressure factors for concern. But experts are beginning to look at alternative anxiety treatments.

A lot of the studies that do exist have centered on pressure factors for nervousness before a potentially stressful situation or surgical procedure, rather than general stress.

For instance, *a 2015 overview of several studies examining the consequences of acupressure on anxiety discovered that acupressure appeared to help relieve stress before a surgical procedure such as surgery.*

Another 2015 research of 85 people hospitalized for malignancy treatment discovered that acupressure helped to lessen their anxiety.

A 2016 study viewed anxiety in 77 students with severe menstrual pain. Acupressure applied at the fantastic surge pressure point during three menstrual cycles reduced stress in research participants by the finish of the 3rd cycle.

A 2018 research discovered that acupressure helped reduce anxiety and stress symptoms in women getting fertility treatments.

Much larger studies saw a need to have a firm grip on how to use pressure factors for anxiety. However, the existing studies haven't found any unwanted effects of acupressure on panic symptoms, so it might be worth a go if you're seeking to get one of these new approaches.

Just retain in mind that these studies also claim that acupressure appears to provide **temporary** rest from symptoms. Be sure to match all the stress management, therapy, or other treatments recommended by your physician while attempting acupressure.

Know when to see a Medical Expert

While acupressure might provide some short term rest from anxiety symptoms, there's very little proof that it'll assist with long-term anxiety.

If you discover that your anxiety symptoms are developing, which makes it hard to visit work or college or to interfere with your associations, it could be time to speak to a health care provider or therapist — worried about the price of therapy? Listed below are therapy options for each budget.

You should speak to a health care provider or therapist if you begin to experience:

- Emotions of depression.

- Thoughts of suicide.

- Panic attacks.

- Trouble sleeping.

- Headaches.

- digestive problems

Acupuncture for Anxiety Attacks

Complementary and substitute medicine (CAM) is thought of as several unconventional practices and products used to market health and therapeutic. Lately, CAM methods have become popular; to treat mental health issues, including depressive disorder, post-traumatic stress disorder (PTSD), and other anxiousness disorders. Some typically standard CAM procedures include intensifying muscle rest, aromatherapy, yoga exercise, and massage therapy.

Acupuncture is a different type of CAM practice that may enhance personal wellbeing. Considered one of the very most popular types of CAM, acupuncture happens to be being used to take care of an array of conditions. As acupuncture is growing in recognition, more research has been centered on this treatment for the freak out symptoms.

What's Acupuncture?

Acupuncture is a recovery technique that originated a large number of years back from traditional Chinese language medication (TCM). This practice is dependent on the idea that an imbalance in energy triggers medical ailments and mental health disorders. TCM theorizes proves that your body contains essential life energy called chi; when your body and brain are working correctly, chi should move through the body's energy stations. These stations are called meridians and can be found at certain factors throughout your body. According to the custom, sometimes chi becomes congested in various meridian pathways, resulting in disease or disorders.

The purpose of acupuncture is to revive the medical and balance of the channels. During acupuncture treatment classes, small needles are positioned along with specific parts of the body. Referred to as acupuncture factors, these areas are usually where blockage of energy may be happening. The needles come in several thicknesses and sizes and are accustomed to stimulate and start blocked stations of power.

Until the past due 1990s, acupuncture needles weren't named tools to take care of medical ailments. In 1997, the *U. S. Food and Medication Administration (FDA)* approved the utilization of acupuncture needles as medical devices. Throughout that same 12 months, acupuncture was identified by the Countrywide Institutes of Health (NIH) for treating pain management and other medical ailments. The FDA presently regulates the requirements for acupuncture needle use and security.

Getting Treated with Acupuncture

If you're thinking about treating your panic and anxiety symptoms through acupuncture, consult your physician; you must get these services from a certified acupuncturist. Professional acupuncture partitioners can be located through websites, like the Countrywide Certification Commission rate for Acupuncture and Oriental Medication and the American Academy of Medical Acupuncture. The usage of acupuncture to take care of medical and mental health issues continues to go up, which makes it more readily available; because it has been examined for effectiveness, and it is available through many hospitals; some plans may cover a few of your acupuncture treatments.

Clinical trials examining acupuncture for anxiety show some excellent results. However, this research has many restrictions, including small test sizes and limited ways to measure results. Acupuncturists and doctors are unclear about why it can help with stress and anxiety, but research has mentioned that acupuncture seems to have a calming impact. More rigorous clinical tests have to be conducted to be able to prove the potency of acupuncture for nervousness disorders.

Not absolutely all CAM practices have been thoroughly researched for protection and effectiveness; more info on the medical evidence, basic safety, and risks of varied CAM practices are available at the *Countrywide Middle for Complementary and Alternative Medication website.* More standard treatment plans for anxiety attacks, such as medications and psychotherapy, have been more backed by research. However, acupuncture may be considered a helpful addition to your standard treatment solution. Acupuncture may be the excess treatment you will need in reducing stress, stress, and anxiety attacks symptoms.

The 5 Best Acupuncture Factors for Anxiety

Nothing diminishes panic faster than an action quote; there are a large number of acupuncture factors for anxiety. Stress can be treated with an enormous selection of acupuncture point combinations predicated on the root pattern, which is exclusive to each individual. However, these five acupuncture factors for anxiousness represent the ones I take advantage of most in my clinic; based on your unique symptoms and encounters as a person, your treatment changes. These factors will help your stress and anxiety and will likely differ from treatment to treatment as your symptoms change.

Acupuncture factors help treats nervousness by activating the nervous system, specifically the parasympathetic nervous system, which reduces cortisol stress hormones. Acupuncture also produces endorphins, natural pain-killing opioids, and other feel-good chemicals in mind. Chronic stress creates deep neural pathways that may be hard to improve. By spending 1-2 hours every week in circumstances of rest, you are assisting in creating a new neural pathway and stopping reinforcing the panic tract. Medications for anxiousness tend to be highly addictive and also have dangerous drawbacks symptoms, such as severe rebound stress and anxiety.

Acupuncture can perform long-lasting results without adverse part effects.

1. Heart 7

This point is situated on the *ulnar side of the wrist* and works to calm the Shen, or "spirit." Whenever we have repressed feelings or sleepless evenings, or even if we desire vividly we might come with an imbalance called *"Heart Open fire" in Traditional Chinese language Medication*; other symptoms of centerfire including, race center, palpitations or center flutters, sweating during the night, high blood circulation pressure, red-tipped tongue, and red face. This imbalance is treated by calming the center, which Centre 7 does superbly.

2. Regulating Vessel 24du 20 and du 24 acupuncture factors for anxiety

This point is situated just *within the hairline in the heart of the forehead*. It works to relax the anxious system by sending energy down.

Race thoughts and "monkey brain" make it hard to relax, which acupuncture points helps immediately that anxious energy down and out.

3. *Pericardium 6*

This point is situated within the *wrist, about 3 inches from the crease.* It is accessible for assisting with nausea and lots of the magnetic bracelets sold for car and sea sickness work by stimulating this aspect. Furthermore, to deal with nausea, this aspect opens the upper body and the center. The pericardium is the protector of the center, and sometimes whenever we are stressed, we are overprotected and guarded. This aspect counteracts the contracting energy of nervousness.

Shenmen acupuncture factors for anxiety4.

4. *Shenmen*

This aspect is positioned *in the ear*; ear factors might appear scary; however, they are very relaxing; this aspect calms the soul by helping your body change into parasympathetic or "rest and break down" mode. As opposed to "battle or airline flight" setting, activating the parasympathetic system causes cortisol stress hormones to drop, reducing anxiety. Ear factors easily access the central anxious system as the nerves go to the brain center.

Yintang acupuncture factors for anxiety

5. *Yintang*

The best of the acupuncture points for anxiety is located between *your brows*. In Hinduism and yoga exercises, this is known as the third vision; this area is situated on the pineal gland, which helps control melatonin. Melatonin is a hormone accountable for restful rest and healthy rest/wake cycles; this aspect is uniquely powerful at dealing with insomnia, caused by overthinking.

Chapter 3

The Acupuncture Factors for Legs

Chinese medicine theory believes your body's energy, or qi, circulates through energy channels called **meridians**. These meridians match the internal organs, which are considered to govern their energy stream; several meridians run the distance of the legs, the belly, spleen, gallbladder, kidney, and liver organ channels; stimulating several points to make a difference in lowering the leg health. Pain, weakness, and numbness may be affected by needling or pressing specific calf points.

Acupuncture

What to find out about an Acupuncture Appointment;

Speak to your doctor before trying acupuncture, especially if you have medical ailments that impact your circulatory and nervous systems. A certified acupuncturist will start by requesting about your health background, collecting current and past information to produce a Chinese medication diagnosis; she will also ask to check out your tongue, take your pulse on both wrists and discuss her meant treatment solution; thin needles will be put into various places, and leave set for between 10 and 45 minutes. During this period, you can relax and meditate while hearing music, or even rest. If you might feel instant results, several or even more sessions are usually recommended to manage your conditions properly.

Meridians on the Legs

Energy meridians run along the back and edges of your legs, surrounding your leg and ankle bones, as well as getting to your toes; it can be indicated for local treatment dysfunctions within the region surrounding the idea. Besides, they serve other functions, such as alleviating pain, numbness and bloating, increasing energy, or balancing feelings. The spleen route can impact muscle power, quality of bloodstream, and bloat. Belly meridian factors can move energy blocks and relieve pain, while kidney factors can increase energy and reduce warmth; the liver organ and gallbladder stations inspire feelings like anger, bloodstream disorders, and menstrual problems.

Factors Responsible for Pain or Swelling

For pain and swelling of the legs, your practitioner may choose kidney point 1, spleen 6, gallbladder 40 and 41 or liver organ 3. Kidney 1 is situated on every single foot, helping restore essential strength and energy while reducing pain and bloating. Gallbladder 40 and 41 pass on power, concentrating on pain in the hips and calves. Spleen 6 can help regulate dampness, resolving bloating around the inner ankle joint area.

Numbness and Weakness

Numbness and weakness in the hip and legs can be regulated by stimulating gallbladder factors 29 and 31, as well as abdomen 33 and 37, kidney 1 and 9, and bladder 40 or 58. Situated in the hip are the outer thigh and leading thigh areas, respectively, gallbladder 29, 31, and tummy 33 are indicated for numbness or weakness in the low extremities. Kidney 9 and belly 37 are located on the weak knee, while bladder 40 and 58 are located near the back again of the leg and leg, respectively. Each one of these points can relieve pain, numbness, and weakness in the hip and legs.

Acupuncture & Hormone Balance

Although acupuncture might not seem just like a reasonable choice for hormonal imbalances, it could involve some benefits. Acupuncture is part of traditional Chinese language medication TCM, which consists of inserting slim needles into specific factors of the body. The elements match different organs whose energy operates along with stations called meridians. Regarding TCM theory, stimulating factors can help restore healthy balance to the body. Speak to your doctor about acupuncture; find a professional Chinese language practitioner to go over your hormonal balance.

Inserting Acupuncture Needles

Hormones

Hormones play essential roles in a vast selection of functions within you, including metabolism, duplication, and sleep-wake cycles. Relating to traditional western medical technology, hormones are secreted by glands in the human brain and body, like the pituitary and adrenal glands; they travel via the bloodstream to various cells to execute their jobs. Although much emphasis is positioned on sex hormones like estrogen and testosterone, thyroid and adrenal hormones are just like crucial to ideal health.

Chinese Theory

Acupuncture.com says that Chinese medication considers hormones to be always a part of a person's Jing, or substance. You are given birth to a degree of life pressure, or fact, which is stored in your kidney, and used during your lifetime to nourish cells, cells, and organs. Jing includes blood and liquids, and yang, which include energy and warmness. Based on the website, when substance depletes, its experience is similar to hormonal imbalances, such as menopause or impotence; Chinese language medicine treatments concentrate on factors that can restore fact; organs like the kidneys and the liver organ are also involved with hormone balance.

Kidney

In "A Manual of Acupuncture" by *Peter Deadman*, the kidney is referred to as being the foundation of life within you. It stores your substance and dominates duplication, development, and development. Because Traditional western medication believes hormones to try out a huge role in these procedures, your Chinese specialist can include kidney acupuncture factors in your hormone-balancing treatment. In March 2010, the *"Journal of Traditional Chinese language Medicine"* featured a report that investigated the consequences of specific acupuncture point activation on the reproductive hormone gonadotropin-releasing hormone. The analysis discovered that the kidney's energy collection, or meridian, performed a job in stimulating the discharge of the hormone; kidney point 10 experienced a significant influence on release.

Liver/Gallbladder

The liver organ and gallbladder is a pair of yin-yang, according to Chinese medicine theory as the yin body organ, the liver organ stores and keeps bloodstream and governs a woman's menstrual period; the gallbladder excretes yang action bile for the breakdown of food. The analysis in the *"Journal of Traditional Chinese Medication"* also lists gallbladder and liver organ points as positively revitalizing the release of gonadotropin-releasing hormone. Gallbladder factors 26 and 34, as well as liver organ points 14, were outlined.

Ren/Du Channels

The ren route is also known as the conception vessel, relating to *Deadman's publication*, whose factors work to harmonize disorders in their geographic area. The route works along the midline of leading of your body, and it is often used to take care of infertility of women and men, and assist in menopausal issues. The du route, known as the regulating vessel, moves along the midline of the trunk of your body; "*A Manual of Acupuncture*" claims it mediates between your brain and the center. In conditions of reproductive hormone excitement, conception vessel factors four and 17 were detailed in the analysis in "*Journal of Traditional Chinese Medication*," along with regulating vessel three.

Chapter 4

Cluster Headaches

Cluster headaches are some relatively brief but excruciating headaches every day for a week or weeks at the same time; you tend to get them at precisely the same time each year, like the springtime or fall. For their seasonal character, people often mistake cluster headaches for symptoms of allergies or business stress.

We have no idea what can cause them, but we can say for sure a nerve in that person is involved, creating extreme pain around one of your eyes. It's so awful that a lot of people can't sit down still and can often speed during an assault. Cluster headaches can become more severe when compared to a migraine; however, they usually don't last for that long.

These are minimal common kinds of headaches, affecting significantly less than 1 in 1,000 people. Men have them more than women do; you usually start to get them before age group 30. Cluster headaches may vanish completely (get into remission) for a few months or years; however, they can come back again without any caution.

What Happens

You get a cluster headache whenever a specific nerve pathway in the human brain is activated; that transmission seems to result from a deeper area of the brain called the hypothalamus, where, in fact, the "internal natural clock" that handles your rest and wake cycles lives.

The nerve that is affected is known as the trigeminal nerve, and it's accountable for sensations such as temperature or pain in that person. It's near your eyesight, and its branches up to your forehead, across your cheek, down your jaw range, and above your hearing on a single side, too. A root brain condition, like a tumor or aneurysm, won't cause these headaches.

Characteristics of Cluster Headaches

Many things make this kind of headache different. They include:

- **Velocity:** Cluster headaches generally reach their

full push quickly; within 5 or 10 minutes.

- **Pain:** It's more often than not, one-sided, and it remains on a single side throughout a period, enough time if you are getting daily episodes. Whenever a new headaches period starts, it could switch to the contrary part, but that's uncommon; it might be throbbing or constant. You'll feel it behind or on one eye; it could pass on to your forehead, temple, nasal area, cheek, or top gum on that aspect, your head may be sensitive, you could feel your bloodstream pulsing.

- **Brief duration:** Cluster headaches usually only last 30 to 90 minutes; they could be as short as quarter-hour or as long as 3 hours, but they disappear. You will most probably get someone who experiences one of three of the headaches each day, but some individuals have only one almost every other day, while some have them up to 8 times per day.

- **Predictable:** Attacks appear to be from the circadian rhythm, your 24-hour clock. They happen so regularly, generally at the same time every day, they are called "noisy alarms headaches." They could even wake you up a couple of hours after you go to sleep. Nighttime episodes can become more severe than daytime ones.

- **Frequent:** A lot of people are sure to get daily headaches for 14 days to three months; among these periods, they will be pain-free for at least 14 days.

Symptoms

The pain usually starts suddenly. When that occurs, you might notice:

- Pain or a mild burning up sensation.

- Swollen or drooping eye.

- Smaller pupil in the attention.

- Eye inflammation or watering.

- Runny or congested nose.

- Red and warm face.

- Sweating.

- You're private to light

Cluster headaches are more prevalent in people who smoke or are heavy drinkers. Throughout a cluster period, you will be more delicate to alcoholic beverages and nicotine; just little alcoholic beverages can result in headaches.

Possible Causes and Triggers

When you're in the center of a cluster period, these can bring on the headache:

- Cigarette smoke.

- Alcohol.

- Strong smells

Treatment

You have several options as it pertains to treating these headaches

Medications

- ***Acute stroke treatments***: This helps when the headaches hit.

- ***Triptans***: These drugs are one of the better ways to take care of the pain. You can find:

Sumatriptan (Alsuma, Imitrex, Sumavel), which works both as a go or inhaled

Zolmitriptan (Zomig)

Dihydroergotamine (D.H.E. 45): This prescription drug is dependent on the ergot fungus.

- ***Lidocaine***: This is a pain reliever, utilizing a nose spray.

- ***Oxygen***: Your physician might call it inhaled oxygen. You'll breathe it in through a nose and mouth mask for a quarter-hour.

Preventive medicine could stop a headache before it starts, your physician can prescribe medication to shorten the space of the cluster as well as lessen the severe nature of your attacks, including:

- *Corticosteroid, like prednisone, for a short while.*

- *Sodium (Depakene, Depakote).*

- *Ergotamine tartrate (Cafergot, Ergomar).*

- *Gabapentin.*

- *Carbonate*

- *Topiramate (Qudexy XR, Topamax, Trokendi XR)*

- *Verapamil (Calan, Covera, Verelan)*

<u>Occipital nerve stop (your physician could also call it occipital nerve injection)</u>: The physician will inject a variety of anesthetic and steroids into these nerves. Located at the bottom of your skull, they're usually the starting place for headaches; that is a short-term treatment until a precautionary can begin to work.

Nerve Activation: Some individuals who don't react to medication have better fortune with:

<u>Occipital nerve stimulation</u>: Your physician surgically implants a tool that sends electric impulses to the band of nerves at the bottom of your skull.

Neuromodulator: These FDA-approved non-invasive devices include:

Cefaly: You put electrodes on your forehead and connect these to a headband-like controller that sends indicators to your supraorbital nerve.

Gamma-Core: This device, also called a non-invasive vague nerve stimulator (NVNS), uses electrodes to send indicators to the nerve.

Surgery

If nothing else works, surgery may be a choice for individuals who do not get a rest from cluster headaches. Deep brain stimulation that involves putting an electrode deep in the brain is losing opt to less invasive options.

Most methods involve blocking the trigeminal nerve, a primary pathway for pain. It settings the region around your eyes, but a misstep can cost weakness in your jaw and lack of feeling in that person and head.

Lifestyle Changes

These moves will help you avoid cluster headaches:

Keep a regular sleep plan: A significant change to your program can start a headache.

Skip alcoholic beverages: Any type, even ale, and wines can trigger an episode of headaches when you're in a cluster series.

Alternative Treatments

Capsaicin: A nose spray of the pain reliever will help.

Melatonin: This medication, known for easing sleep issues like aircraft lag, might lower the number of headaches.

Chapter 5

How to use Pressure Factors to alleviate Headaches

There are a few popular pressure points in the torso thought to relieve headaches. Here's where they may be and ways to utilize them:

Union valley

The union valley points can be found on the internet in the middle of your thumb and index finger. To take care of headaches:

- Begin by pinching this area with the thumb and index finger of your reverse hands firmly - however, not painfully - for 10 seconds.

- Next, make small circles with your thumb upon this area in a single direction for ten mere seconds each.

- Continue doing this process on the Union Valley point on your contrary hand.

This sort of pressure point treatment is thought to relieve tension in the top and neck. The pressure is often associated with headaches.

Drilling bamboo

Drilling bamboo factors can be found at the indentations on either aspect of the location where the bridge of your nose area matches the ridge of your eyebrows. To use these pressure factors to treat headaches:

- Use both of your index hands to apply company pressure to both elements at once.

- Keep for 10 seconds.

- Release and do it again.

Coming in contact with these pressure factors can relieve headaches that are triggered by eye strain and sinus pain or pressure.

Gates of consciousness

The gates of consciousness pressure points can be found at the *bottom of the skull in the parallel hollow areas between your two vertical neck muscles.* To use these pressure factors:

- Place your index and middle hands of either hand onto these pressure factors.

- Press firmly upward on both edges simultaneously for ten mere seconds, then release and do it again

- Applying strong touch to these pressure factors can help reduce headaches triggered by tension in the neck.

Third eye

The Third eye point is available in the middle of your two eyebrows, where the bridge of your nose meets your forehead.

Utilize the index finger of 1 hand to use firm pressure to the area for 1 minute.

Firm pressure put on the third attention pressure point is considered to relieve eyestrain and sinus pressure that often causes headaches.

Shoulder well

The shoulder well is situated at the *edge of your shoulder*, halfway in the middle of your shoulder point and the bottom of your neck. To utilize th is pressure point:

- Utilize the thumb of 1 hand to use firm, round pressure up to now for 1 minute.

- Then change and repeat on the contrary side.

- Applying solid touch to the make well pressure point can help alleviate stiffness in your neck

Chapter 6

Acupuncture for Digestive Problems

Published July 18, 2017, by Hailin Wu, OM Clinical / Faculty Supervisor, Program Director & filed under Acupuncture and Massage College.

Acupuncture for digestive problems is an effective and safe way to naturally treat many acute and chronic conditions of the vital body. If you've attempted conventional medication to keep digestive issues in balance without success, consider acupuncture, which is an alternative health treatment without part effects.

Acupuncture can assist in treating many digestion disorders, including:

- Bacterial infections.

- Peptic ulcers.

- Heartburn.

- Lactose intolerance.

- Gastrointestinal tract bleeding.

- Inflammatory conditions.

- Hiatus hernia syndrome

So how exactly does acupuncture treatment help?

Using acupuncture for digestive problems functions by nourishing related organs, reducing irritation of the belly and pancreas, and enhancing digestive functions. Throughout treatment, the specialist will identify certain acupuncture factors on your body, typically the ones that speed metabolism, increase gastrointestinal muscle contraction and rest, reduce gastric acid secretion, and control small and large intestine function, and restores abdomen acidity on track levels.

Together with Chinese language herbal medicine and stress reduction techniques, acupuncture for digestive problems is useful in treating general gastrointestinal symptoms.

Furthermore, to acupuncture for digestive problems,

moxibustion - a method of applying the herb mugwort to acupuncture factors - can also be utilized as an anti-inflammatory agent and also to notify imbalances. Individuals often experience long-term symptomatic comfort with acupuncture for digestive problems, as well as reduced stress and improved energy.

Acupuncture for digestive problems may integrate suggestions for lifestyle modifications to be able to correct diet imbalances and regulate digestive function. The World Health Corporation identifies acupuncture for digestive issues as a highly effective treatment for digestive imbalance.

The Sources of Digestive Disorders

Digestion disorders may be the effect of a variety of factors, such as chronic stress and other nutritional issues, such as overeating or eating way too many high-fat foods. Acupuncture can treat digestive imbalance by reducing stress and regulating the endocrine and anxious system hyperactivity that often accompanies digestive disorder patterns.

Acupuncture is a cure that can be built-into allopathic or holistic health care seamlessly. Acupuncture for digestive problems is an all-natural health maintenance therapy.

Acupuncture and Abdomen Disorders

I am often asked this question whenever a conversation arises about tummy disorders and acupuncture; "can acupuncture help me personally to avoid needing antacids regularly?" or "how about my acid reflux?"

Folks are amazed once I clarify to them that acupuncture can treat most gastrointestinal issues such as acid reflux disorder, bloating, and indigestion very effectively.

According to Chinese language Medicine, the Belly is a significant official (organ) inside our body. It is so essential that there surely is a custom of acupuncture that concentrates mainly on the Tummy (and its own 'sister body organ' the Spleen). If the Belly cannot function to its fullest capacity when compared to a person who struggles to be wholly nourished in their Body, Brain, or Spirit.

The Stomach is essential for getting our food nourishment (or GuQi) and also our mental and spirit level nourishment. We have to process information (i.e., what we should read, study, listen to, see, etc.) which work consists of our belly. We also need to receive and process psychological materials, which also involves our abdomen.

A lot of my patients who are in university or graduate frequently have Stomach issues, which have mostly resolved with acupuncture and vanished after they complete their studies. I've treated many people who have medical diagnoses of acid reflux disorder or acid reflux; these conditions, along with problems like belching, hiccupping, nausea, and even throwing up, are categorized as the group of Rebellious Stomach Qi. When the Stomach becomes weakened or stressed or out of balance the Qi may rise, which leads to the symptoms mentioned above (rebellious Stomach). You will find multiple points and treatment possibilities to take care of stomach disorders. Remember, the Stomach is one of the most extended meridians on your body; they have 45 points onto it. Combine that with the interplay of other 'Officials' on your body (as I'll elaborate below), and an acupuncturist will come up with multiple treatment plans for you.

Many fundamental imbalances in the torso can result in 'rebellious stomach qi.' For instance, the Liver Standard (or meridian) is accountable for the clean flow of feelings (according to Chinese medicine). Whenever we are chronically stressed or tense/anxious/angry/ depressed, etc., our Liver Official may start to impact onto the Stomach leading to the Stomach to 'rebel.' Just how many times perhaps you have heard someone cry 'I can't stomach it anymore' they could lose their appetite. Some individuals may gain in appetite.

Another cause could be related to the Kidney Recognized (or meridian). Regarding Chinese Medication, one of the items the Kidney does is help warm the organs to allow them to function optimally. Sometimes, with age, the Kidney Official weakens and has less capacity to warm your body; this may cause the Stomach to decline response. I'm sure you have heard about older people complaining of more difficulty in digesting different kinds of food auspices as they age. Or, they can no more eat large meals- when smaller, more frequent meals are better tolerated.

Many people complain of a far more generalized symptom of 'sensitive stomach.' They present with bloating and gas, making their waistbands feel tight after meals. Often these folks report an extremely long history of the symptoms. Once in order, the sign may occasionally arrive when they are extremely stressed about something in their life. Or it becomes their 'check engine light' reminding them that they have to practice a few of the new coping strategies they've learned in their acupuncture journey. The symptom has resolved to the stage where it's the exception as opposed to the rule in their life. Quite simply, acupuncture has helped them to access the central point where they can manage their stomach rather than it controlling them.

Did you know the belly functions at its best whenever we take in warm food; iced drinks, cold foods, freezing desserts, actually stress the stomach, food that is too spicy can also put pressure on the stomach as time passes. Our diet plan over our lifetime can eventually donate to the weakening of our stomach once we age. An acupuncturist is trained to help identify what's stressing your stomach so that changes in lifestyle can be suggested.

As well as the history you provide to your acupuncturist, the pulse reading and the tongue evaluation offer valuable information in identifying the health of your stomach. This can help in formulating a cure plan that is designed for you.

Keep your Belly at heart when you take in meals. It doesn't like being overly stuffed, which burdens the Abdomen. So, eat slower, laugh a lot, take smaller portions, don't drink cold beverages with your meal (sip on room temperature water instead), and eat during the day.

Chapter 7

Acupuncture for Lowering High Blood Pressure

On the 11th of June 2001, some individuals swear by acupuncture; they said pincushion healed bad migraine headaches or relentless back again pain, others remain skeptical, dismissing the historical practice as mumbo jumbo. Now, researchers have started investigating the activities in cardiovascular disease, and they have found out not just that acupuncture works, but why and exactly how. They once informed WebMD that blood circulation pressure medication might be replaced with a few pins and needles.

John C. Longhurst, MD, Ph.D., "I met an investigator who'd been carrying out work in acupuncture for a long time. I noticed that he was a good scientist," he says. "I, like the majority of researchers, thought acupuncture was a great deal of hocus pocus. However, when I noticed his work, I understood there is something to it."

Long Hurst, a teacher of medication at the university or college of California, Irvine, University of Medicine, started four investigations into the underlying systems of acupuncture; in it, his team tested cats with cardiovascular disease. He said, "we demonstrated that acupuncture helped the pets by reducing ischemia, having less air to the center" triggered when arteries are blocked; that was hard proof that the treatment worked well. Next, they attempted to regulate how it was occurring.

Long Hurst says in acupuncture, the unseen pathways connecting one body part to some other are called meridians. "They can be found over major [nerve] pathways that are accessed when you put a needle in." Rousing the pathway "sends impulses to the mind, activating different areas." Some influence pain, "which is why acupuncture can control pain," he says, "as well as others regulate the heart."

One particular area, right above the spinal cord in the mind stem, regulates the release of adrenaline, a chemical substance that makes the heart pound and blood circulation pressure soar. However, when they induced, adrenaline hurry in pets, and acupuncture avoided this from taking place. It blocked the result," says Long Hurst. Hearts defeat usually, and blood circulation pressure remained low.

In the 3rd study, the team found they could invert acupuncture's heart-healthy effects by injecting cats with a synthetic version of naturally occurring opioids -- brain chemicals that create a "runner's high," kicking in when we're in severe pain. "So, we're narrowing it down, getting ultimately more specific and comprehensive in conditions of what's happening," says Long Hurst.

Fourth research is underway in human being topics, he tells WebMD, but it's still premature to attract any conclusions. The best goal of the work is to help the large numbers of patients with ischemia, high blood circulation pressure, and irregular pulse, or heart arrhythmias, he tells WebMD. "The existing meds have a lot of side results; if we can reduce [their medication needed] with acupuncture, which might be great."

Experts agree it isn't a far-fetched idea. "There need to be something more to acupuncture than the placebo impact of hypnosis," says Joseph Alpert, MD, Flinn Teacher of Medication and chairman of the division of medication at the College or university of Az in Tucson. "My co-workers have seen folks have opened up center surgery with only acupuncture, no anesthesia; this isn't a couple of malarkey," he tells WebMD, "it's real."

Pascal J. Goldschmidt, MD, FACC, principal of cardiology at Duke School, agrees that "It isn't an accident that individuals have been doing acupuncture for such a long time," he tells WebMD. The results are "fairly clear that it is not a placebo impact. Acupuncture appears to be having a comparatively specific influence on the control of blood circulation pressure."

Acupuncture and Stroke

Strokes can occur to anyone from delivery through adulthood. There are two different kinds of strokes; a stroke that occurs when blood circulation is no more travelling the mind is named an *ischemic heart stroke*. A stroke that occurs when a bloodstream vessel breaks or leaks in mind is called a *hemorrhagic heart stroke*. Both types of stroke are severe and, concerning the severity, can cause long term damage; rehabilitation can be an essential part of dealing with a heart stroke. As you could expect, rehabilitation options are enormous and cover from exercise to cognitive and psychological activities.

Some see acupuncture as a match to traditional treatment methods. Continue reading to get more on the benefits and dangers of getting acupuncture after a heart stroke.

What are the medical advantages of acupuncture?

Benefits

- Acupuncture is a widely accepted alternative treatment for chronic pain.

- It's also used to relax your body and mind.

Acupuncture is a Chinese language healing practice that is around for years; it involves the utilization of slim, disinfected needles placed into the epidermis by a qualified acupuncturist. These needles are positioned in specific parts of the body that are thought to unleash different types of all-natural curing energy. For instance, applying pressure to the "third vision point" between your eyebrows is believed to relieve headaches pain.

Although acupuncture is mainly recognized as an all-natural treatment for chronic pain, its potential benefits extend much beyond that; it's been used to assist in improving sleeping patterns and digestive function. The practice, also, has been thought to relax your brain and reduce stress or panic.

What does the study say?

In a single 2005 research, people who had experienced a stroke received the opportunity to try acupuncture therapy. The purpose of the treatment was to help decrease pain and discomfort because of the stroke. Experts found that individuals who received acupuncture noticed an improvement in wrist spasticity and flexibility in the wrist and make. Although people who received acupuncture do see more development in comparison with those who didn't receive acupuncture, the amount of improvement wasn't considered medically significant.

Far more recent research shows that acupuncture coupled with exercise can succeed against make pain caused by stroke.

More research is essential to determine whether acupuncture has a definitive influence on recovery from stroke.

So how exactly does acupuncture work?

At the appointment, your acupuncturist will review your trouble and discuss the way they believe they will help you. Typically, they'll take a look at your tongue for more info about your wellbeing and take your pulse.

When it's time for the procedure, they'll ask you lay down; with regards to the area your acupuncturist will treat, you might be face up, face down, or working for you. Your acupuncturist will softly put in sterile, single-use needles in the areas they believe the body will take advantage of the most.

You'll likely feel them inserting the needles; nevertheless, you probably won't feel any pain. During this period, your acupuncturist may add high temperatures or therapeutic massage to your therapy.

One program typically lasts thirty minutes. A typical span of acupuncture therapy requires up to 12 classes. Some insurance firms cover the expense of acupuncture therapy, so make sure to consult with your supplier about your alternatives.

Dangers and Warnings

Risks

- The usage of unsterilized needles can cause health complications.

- You might experience bruising or bleeding across the injection sites.

Before seeing an acupuncturist, visit your physician and discuss your desire to include acupuncture to your recovery plan. They can help you evaluate whether this is the most suitable choice for you. Acupuncture might not be for you if you have a blood loss disorder or if you're taking bloodstream thinners.

After consulting your physician, research acupuncturists locally; ensure that they're certified and pursuing all health rules.

After your appointment, you might experience blood loss, bruising, or soreness at the insertion sites. That is a standard response to the procedure. If you start experiencing any uncommon symptoms, you should seek advice from your doctor.

Alternatives to Acupuncture

If you're not an applicant for acupuncture or want to try traditional ways of treatment, you have a great many other options. Based on your needs, you might receive inpatient or outpatient treatment. This might include conversation, occupational, and physical therapy. These treatments can help you to regain the utilization of your talk, as well as the number of movements in your hands, hip and legs, and hands.

If the human brain was damaged throughout your stroke, you might even need to visit a neurologist for even more treatment. It could also be beneficial to consult with a psychiatrist. They can help you sort out your emotions as you navigate your recovery.

Chapter 8

Health Advantages of Hearing Acupuncture

Hearing acupuncture is a kind of acupuncture that involves inserting needles into specific parts of the ear; revitalizing these factors is considered to promote curing in the areas of your body. Generally known as auricular therapy or auricular-acupuncture, ear acupuncture is often incorporated into standard acupuncture treatments.

Although ear acupuncture is predicated on the principles of traditional Chinese language medicine (a kind of alternative medicine that started in China), it originated in the middle-20th century by *French scientist Paul Nogier*.

Uses

Ear acupuncture is utilized to enhance the body's circulation of vital energy (also called chi or qi) and even to restore the equilibrium between yin and yang (two opposing but complementary energies) within the inner organs. In traditional Chinese medicine, each one of these results is known as essential in dealing with disease and attaining health.

In alternative medicine, ear acupuncture is usually used for these and other health issues:

- Allergies.//
- Anxiety.
- Arthritis.
- Chronic pain.
- Constipation.
- Depression.
- Fibromyalgia.
- Headaches.
- Insomnia.
- Irritable bowel syndrome.

- Low back again, pain.

- Migraines

Furthermore, ear acupuncture may also be used to improve mood, assist in smoking cessation, alleviate pain, promote sounder rest, relieve stress, and support weight loss.

Benefits

Although large-scale medical trials on ear acupuncture are lacking, lots of studies claim that this therapy may assist in treating several health conditions. Here are several findings on ear acupuncture and its potential health advantages.

Insomnia

Several studies indicate that ear acupuncture can help relieve insomnia. These studies supported a released in *Complementary Therapies in Medication in 2003*, which tested the consequences of a kind of ear acupuncture, which involves using magnetic pearls to stimulate acupuncture points.

For the analysis, 15 seniors with insomnia were treated with hearing acupuncture for three weeks. Results exposed that individuals experienced a substantial increase in both quality and level of rest, with improvements enduring for half a year after treatment ended.

Smoking

Research on ear acupuncture's effectiveness as a smoking cessation help has yielded combined results within a 2004 study released in *the Swiss Journal of Research in Complementary and Natural Classical Medicine*; for instance, *a survey of 126 people who had undergone ear acupuncture for smoking cessation discovered that the procedure had a one-year success rate of 41.1%.* Based on the study's authors, this success rate makes hearing acupuncture "a competitive option to orthodox remedies withdrawal methods."

In a report published in the Journal of *the American Board of Family Medicine*, however, a trial involving 125 people discovered that ear acupuncture was more effective than placebo treatment in enhancing the pace of smoking cessation. The analysis included five consecutive weeks of once-a-week treatments.

Migraines

Ear canal acupuncture may be useful in treating migraines, according to a report published in *Acupuncture & Electro-Therapeutics Research in 2012.* Analyzing findings on 35 migraine patients, the study's author determined that eight weeks of weekly ear acupuncture treatments resulted in significant improvements in pain and mood.

Post-Surgery Pain

For a written report published in *the Journal of Alternative and Complementary Medicine this year 2010*, investigators sized up 17 studies on hearing acupuncture's performance in pain management. The report's authors figured ear acupuncture might succeed in treating different types of pain, especially postoperative pain.

Constipation

Study review posted in *the Journal of Alternative and*

Complementary Medicine this year 2010 shows that ear acupuncture may assist in treating constipation; for the review, researchers examined 29 studies on the utilization of ear acupuncture in constipation management.

Although all the studies reported that ear acupuncture was effective in treating constipation, the author review that due to significant flaws in the reviewed studies, more research is required to confirm these findings.

Using Hearing Acupuncture for Health

If you are considering trying hearing acupuncture, be sure to consult a medical doctor first. Self-treating and avoiding standard care can have serious consequences.

www.ingramcontent.com/pod-product-compliance
Lightning Source LLC
Chambersburg PA
CBHW071123030426
42336CB00013BA/2177